ERYTHROMYCIN STEP TO STEP MANUAL BOOK

Learn the basic things should know before using erythromycin for infections

CHRIS ALDERBALT

Contents

Chapter1 3

   Uses of Erythromycin....................3

Chapter2 21

   Precautions and Warnings of Erythromycin 21

Chapter3 40

   Interactions of Erythromycin with Other Medications.....................40

   The end 60

Chapter1

Uses of Erythromycin

Erythromycin is a broad-spectrum antibiotic that belongs to the macrolide class. It is derived from the bacterium *Saccharopolyspora erythraea* and is known for its ability to treat a wide range of bacterial infections by inhibiting bacterial protein synthesis. Its versatility has made it a go-to option for several types of infections, including respiratory, skin, gastrointestinal, and sexually transmitted infections. Erythromycin also plays an essential role in managing infections caused by atypical bacteria that are resistant to other classes of antibiotics, such as penicillins or cephalosporins.

This antibiotic is favored for its efficacy, especially in patients who may be allergic to penicillin-based antibiotics. Below, we'll explore in detail the various uses of erythromycin, emphasizing how it works in different clinical scenarios, its suitability for certain populations, and its effectiveness against a broad spectrum of pathogens.

Treatment of Respiratory Infections

One of the most common uses of erythromycin is in treating respiratory infections. It is frequently prescribed for bacterial infections affecting the upper and lower respiratory tracts, including conditions like pneumonia, bronchitis, and sinusitis. Erythromycin is particularly effective against respiratory pathogens such as *Streptococcus pneumoniae*, *Haemophilus influenzae*, and *Moraxella catarrhalis*. It is also effective in treating infections caused by atypical bacteria such as *Mycoplasma pneumoniae* and *Legionella pneumophila*.

Pneumonia: Erythromycin is used to treat both typical and atypical pneumonia. Atypical pneumonia, often caused by organisms like *Mycoplasma pneumoniae*, *Chlamydia pneumoniae*, or *Legionella*, is commonly known as "walking pneumonia" because it tends to be less severe than other types. Erythromycin is highly effective against these pathogens, making it a preferred choice in treating atypical pneumonia. In severe cases, erythromycin may be used as part of combination therapy to provide broader coverage against both Gram-positive and Gram-negative bacteria.

Bronchitis and Sinusitis: For patients suffering from bronchitis, especially chronic bronchitis, erythromycin can help alleviate symptoms by targeting the underlying bacterial infection. Similarly, it is useful in cases of bacterial sinusitis, where it works to reduce inflammation and eliminate the bacterial cause of the infection. Erythromycin is often prescribed in these situations when patients are allergic to beta-lactam antibiotics like penicillin.

Skin and Soft Tissue Infections

Erythromycin is widely used to treat skin and soft tissue infections, particularly those caused by Gram-positive bacteria. Infections like impetigo, cellulitis, and erysipelas are commonly treated with erythromycin due to its effectiveness against *Streptococcus* and *Staphylococcus* species.

Impetigo: Impetigo is a superficial bacterial skin infection that primarily affects children. It is commonly caused by *Staphylococcus aureus* or *Streptococcus pyogenes*. Erythromycin is effective in treating mild to moderate cases of impetigo, especially when caused by strains of bacteria that are resistant to penicillin.

Cellulitis and Erysipelas: These are deeper infections that affect the skin and underlying soft tissues. *Streptococcus* species are the most common culprits in cellulitis and erysipelas. Erythromycin works by inhibiting the growth of these bacteria, reducing inflammation, and allowing the immune system to clear the infection. It is especially useful in patients who cannot tolerate penicillin.

Erythromycin is also used to treat **acne vulgaris**, a common skin condition caused by the overgrowth of *Propionibacterium acnes* in the hair follicles. The antibiotic helps reduce the bacterial population on the skin and alleviates the inflammation associated with acne. Though other antibiotics may be more commonly used for acne today, erythromycin remains an option, particularly for patients who have not responded well to other treatments.

Gastrointestinal Infections

Erythromycin is used to treat a variety of gastrointestinal

infections, most notably those caused by *Campylobacter jejuni*, which is a common cause of foodborne illness. Infections from *Campylobacter* can lead to symptoms such as diarrhea, abdominal pain, fever, and nausea, and they are often contracted through contaminated food or water.

Campylobacteriosis: Erythromycin is considered one of the first-line treatments for campylobacteriosis, particularly in severe cases where symptoms are debilitating or when the infection spreads beyond the intestines. Erythromycin helps to clear the infection by stopping the bacteria from replicating, thus speeding up recovery and reducing the risk of complications.

Erythromycin can also be used in the treatment of **gastroparesis**, a condition in which the stomach does not empty food properly due to weakened or uncoordinated muscular contractions. Although this use is not related to its antibiotic properties, erythromycin's ability to stimulate motilin receptors in the gastrointestinal tract can improve gastric motility, making it useful in managing the symptoms of gastroparesis, such as nausea, vomiting, and bloating.

Sexually Transmitted Infections (STIs)

Erythromycin is effective in treating certain sexually transmitted infections (STIs), particularly those caused by bacteria like *Chlamydia trachomatis* and *Treponema pallidum*, the causative agent of syphilis.

Chlamydia: Erythromycin is an alternative treatment for chlamydial infections, particularly in pregnant women who cannot take other antibiotics like doxycycline. Chlamydia infections can affect the genitals, eyes (causing trachoma), or lungs (as in neonatal pneumonia). Erythromycin's ability to target *Chlamydia trachomatis* makes it valuable in preventing complications such as pelvic inflammatory disease (PID) and infertility.

Syphilis: Although penicillin is the primary treatment for syphilis, erythromycin may be used as an alternative in patients who are allergic to penicillin. It is effective in early stages of syphilis by inhibiting the bacteria's protein synthesis and stopping its spread through the body.

Prevention of Neonatal Infections

Erythromycin is commonly used to prevent certain infections in newborns, especially those related to exposure to maternal infections during childbirth. Two major uses include the prevention of eye infections and respiratory infections in newborns.

Ophthalmia Neonatorum: This is a severe eye infection in newborns that can occur when babies are exposed to *Neisseria gonorrhoeae* or *Chlamydia trachomatis* during delivery. Erythromycin is used in newborns to prevent this infection, as it effectively targets both of these bacteria. Preventing ophthalmia neonatorum is critical because the condition can lead to blindness if left untreated.

Neonatal Pneumonia: Infants born to mothers with chlamydia are at risk of developing pneumonia caused by *Chlamydia trachomatis*. Erythromycin is used to treat or prevent this form of neonatal pneumonia, which can be serious and lead to long-term respiratory complications if not managed promptly.

Treatment of Diphtheria and Pertussis

Erythromycin is highly effective in treating **diphtheria**, an infection caused by *Corynebacterium diphtheriae*, and **pertussis** (whooping cough), caused by *Bordetella pertussis*. Both of these infections affect the respiratory system and can be life-threatening, especially in children.

Diphtheria: In cases of diphtheria, erythromycin works by halting the replication of *Corynebacterium diphtheriae*, reducing the spread of the bacteria and preventing the production of toxins that can damage the heart, kidneys, and nervous system. In addition to treating the infection, erythromycin is also used prophylactically in individuals who have been in close contact with a person diagnosed with diphtheria to prevent the spread of the disease.

Pertussis: Whooping cough is a highly contagious respiratory infection that can be severe, especially in infants and young children. Erythromycin is effective in treating pertussis by limiting the replication of *Bordetella pertussis* and reducing the duration and severity of symptoms. It also helps reduce the transmission of the disease to others, making it an important part of public health efforts to control outbreaks.

Use in Patients with Penicillin Allergies

One of the key advantages of erythromycin is its use as an alternative treatment for patients who are allergic to penicillin. Since many bacterial infections that respond to penicillin also respond to erythromycin, it provides an essential treatment option for individuals who cannot tolerate beta-lactam antibiotics. This is particularly important in the treatment of respiratory infections, skin infections, and sexually transmitted infections.

Chapter 2

Precautions and Warnings of Erythromycin

Erythromycin is a widely prescribed macrolide antibiotic used to treat various bacterial infections. While generally considered safe and effective, erythromycin has specific precautions and warnings that both patients and healthcare providers must consider before and during its use. These precautions are essential to prevent adverse reactions, avoid interactions with other medications, and ensure that the drug is used safely, especially in populations that may be more vulnerable to its side effects. Understanding these warnings can help minimize risks and maximize the benefits of erythromycin in treating infections.

1. Allergic Reactions and Hypersensitivity

One of the most important precautions when using erythromycin is the risk of allergic reactions or hypersensitivity. Although allergic reactions are relatively rare, they can occur in some individuals and range from mild to severe. Mild allergic reactions may include symptoms like itching, hives, or rashes. These symptoms generally resolve once the medication is discontinued, but it is crucial to inform a healthcare provider immediately to avoid further complications.

However, more severe allergic reactions, such as anaphylaxis, are a life-threatening concern. Anaphylaxis is a medical emergency characterized by symptoms such as difficulty breathing, swelling of the throat or tongue, rapid heartbeat, dizziness, and a drop in blood pressure. If anaphylaxis occurs, immediate treatment is required, typically involving the administration of epinephrine to counteract the reaction. Patients who have a known allergy to erythromycin or other macrolide antibiotics should avoid using this drug, and it is important that any history of allergies to medications is disclosed to the healthcare provider before starting erythromycin.

2. Liver Function and Hepatic Impairment

Erythromycin is primarily metabolized in the liver, which means it can have a significant impact on liver function. Individuals with pre-existing liver conditions, such as hepatitis, cirrhosis, or fatty liver disease, must take special precautions when using erythromycin. In such patients, the liver may not be able to process the drug efficiently, leading to the accumulation of the medication in the body and increasing the risk of side effects or toxicity.

Erythromycin has been associated with the development of cholestatic hepatitis, a condition where the flow of bile from the liver is obstructed, leading to symptoms like jaundice (yellowing of the skin and eyes), dark urine, light-colored stools, abdominal pain, and fatigue. This condition is usually reversible after discontinuing the medication, but it can become severe if not recognized early.

Patients with liver dysfunction should be closely monitored through regular blood tests to assess liver enzyme levels, and the dosage may need to be adjusted based on the severity of the liver impairment.

3. Cardiac Concerns: QT Prolongation and Arrhythmias

One of the most serious warnings associated with erythromycin is its potential to cause cardiac side effects, particularly in individuals with pre-existing heart conditions. Erythromycin has been shown to prolong the QT interval, which is a specific measurement on an electrocardiogram (ECG) that reflects the time it takes for the heart to reset its electrical activity between beats. QT prolongation can lead to a dangerous type of irregular heartbeat known as *torsades de pointes*, which can result in fainting, seizures, or sudden death if left untreated.

Individuals who are already at risk for QT prolongation, such as those with a family history of long QT syndrome, bradycardia (slow heart rate), or those taking other medications known to affect the heart's electrical system, should use erythromycin with extreme caution. Before prescribing erythromycin, healthcare providers often perform a thorough assessment of the patient's heart function, which may include an ECG. Patients should also be informed about the symptoms of arrhythmias, such as palpitations, dizziness, or fainting, and should seek medical attention immediately if any of these occur while taking erythromycin.

Additionally, certain electrolyte imbalances, particularly low potassium or magnesium levels, can increase the risk of QT prolongation when taking erythromycin. Patients with electrolyte disorders should have these imbalances corrected before starting erythromycin, and their electrolyte levels should be monitored throughout the course of treatment.

4. Drug Interactions

Erythromycin is known to interact with a wide range of other medications, which can increase the risk of side effects or reduce the efficacy of the drugs involved. One of the most significant concerns with erythromycin is its inhibition of certain liver enzymes, particularly the cytochrome P450 (CYP450) system, which is responsible for metabolizing many drugs. By inhibiting these enzymes, erythromycin can cause increased blood levels of medications that are normally metabolized by the CYP450 system, potentially leading to toxicity.

For example, erythromycin can interact with medications used to treat heart conditions, such as calcium channel blockers or antiarrhythmics, increasing the risk of heart-related side effects like QT prolongation. It can also interact with blood thinners, leading to an increased risk of bleeding, or with certain statins, raising the risk of muscle toxicity (rhabdomyolysis).

Patients should provide their healthcare provider with a complete list of all medications they are taking, including over-the-counter drugs and herbal supplements, to avoid potentially dangerous interactions.

5. Gastrointestinal Concerns

While erythromycin is often used to treat bacterial infections in the gastrointestinal tract, it can also cause significant gastrointestinal side effects, including nausea, vomiting, diarrhea, and abdominal pain. These symptoms are common, as erythromycin stimulates motility in the gastrointestinal tract by acting on motilin receptors, which can cause increased contractions of the stomach and intestines.

Patients with pre-existing gastrointestinal conditions, such as irritable bowel syndrome (IBS) or inflammatory bowel disease (IBD), may find that erythromycin exacerbates their symptoms. Additionally, erythromycin has been associated with the development of *pseudomembranous colitis*, a severe form of diarrhea caused by an overgrowth of *Clostridium difficile* (C. difficile). This condition is serious and requires immediate medical attention. Symptoms include watery diarrhea, fever, and severe abdominal pain. In such cases, discontinuation of erythromycin and the initiation of treatment for *C. difficile* are necessary to prevent further complications.

6. Renal Impairment

Although erythromycin is primarily metabolized by the liver, a small portion of the drug is excreted through the kidneys. Patients with renal impairment or chronic kidney disease (CKD) may require dose adjustments to prevent the accumulation of the drug in the body, which could increase the risk of adverse effects. In such cases, healthcare providers typically monitor kidney function through blood tests and adjust the dosage or frequency of erythromycin administration based on the severity of the kidney impairment.

7. Use in Special Populations

Certain populations require extra precautions when using erythromycin due to increased susceptibility to side effects or complications. These populations include pregnant and breastfeeding women, children, and elderly individuals.

Pregnancy and Breastfeeding: Erythromycin is generally considered safe for use during pregnancy, but certain forms of the drug may be associated with an increased risk of adverse effects on the fetus. Pregnant women should consult their healthcare provider to determine whether erythromycin is appropriate for them, and they should only use the medication when the potential benefits outweigh the risks. Erythromycin can pass into breast milk, and while it is usually safe for breastfeeding infants, there is a potential risk of gastrointestinal disturbances or allergic reactions in the nursing baby. Women who are breastfeeding should inform their healthcare provider before starting erythromycin to ensure it is safe for both mother and child.

Children: Erythromycin is commonly prescribed to children for the treatment of infections like respiratory tract infections, ear infections, and skin infections. However, the dosage must be carefully adjusted based on the child's age, weight, and the severity of the infection. Children may also be more prone to certain side effects, such as gastrointestinal upset, and should be monitored for any adverse reactions during treatment.

Elderly Individuals: Older adults may be more susceptible to the side effects of erythromycin, particularly those affecting the liver, kidneys, and heart. Age-related changes in organ function can alter the way the body processes the drug, increasing the risk of toxicity. Additionally, elderly individuals are more likely to be taking multiple medications, raising the potential for drug interactions. Careful monitoring and possible dosage adjustments are often necessary when prescribing erythromycin to older adults.

8. Resistance and Superinfections

Like all antibiotics, erythromycin should be used with caution to prevent the development of antibiotic resistance. Overuse or misuse of antibiotics can lead to the emergence of resistant strains of bacteria, making future infections more difficult to treat. Patients should be advised to take erythromycin exactly as prescribed, complete the full course of the medication even if they feel better, and not use the antibiotic for viral infections, such as the common cold or flu, which it is ineffective against.

In some cases, prolonged use of erythromycin can lead to the development of superinfections, such as fungal infections or infections caused by resistant bacteria. These superinfections occur when the normal balance of microorganisms in the body is disrupted, allowing opportunistic pathogens to grow unchecked. Patients who develop symptoms of a superinfection, such as persistent fever, unusual discharge, or new symptoms during or after treatment, should seek medical advice.

Chapter 3

Interactions of Erythromycin with Other Medications

Erythromycin, a macrolide antibiotic, is widely used for its ability to treat various bacterial infections. While effective in combating numerous bacterial pathogens, erythromycin is known to interact with a broad range of other medications. These interactions can significantly affect the drug's safety and efficacy, sometimes leading to serious consequences, such as increased toxicity, reduced therapeutic effects, or heightened risk of side effects. The potential for erythromycin to interact with other medications arises mainly due to its impact on liver enzymes, particularly the cytochrome P450 (CYP450) system, which is responsible for metabolizing many drugs. Additionally, erythromycin may interact with medications through mechanisms that affect the heart, gastrointestinal system, and other physiological pathways.

Understanding these drug interactions is crucial for healthcare providers to make informed decisions about prescribing erythromycin and for patients to avoid harmful side effects. Below is a comprehensive overview of the most significant interactions of erythromycin with other medications, divided into different categories based on the nature and clinical implications of these interactions.

1. Erythromycin and Cytochrome P450 (CYP450) Enzyme Inhibition

One of the most well-known and clinically significant interactions of erythromycin involves its inhibition of liver enzymes, particularly those within the cytochrome P450 family, specifically the CYP3A4 isoenzyme. The CYP450 system is essential for the metabolism of many drugs, and when erythromycin inhibits these enzymes, it can reduce the clearance of other medications, leading to increased concentrations of these drugs in the bloodstream.

This increase in drug levels can heighten the risk of toxicity and side effects. Drugs that are metabolized by CYP3A4, and therefore may be affected by erythromycin, include a wide variety of medications, such as certain statins, calcium channel blockers, anticonvulsants, and more. The inhibition of CYP3A4 by erythromycin can cause the following drug interactions:

Statins (Cholesterol-Lowering Medications): Erythromycin can interact with statins, particularly those metabolized by CYP3A4, such as simvastatin and atorvastatin. Statins are used to lower cholesterol levels and reduce the risk of cardiovascular diseases. When erythromycin is taken concurrently with statins, it can increase the blood concentration of these drugs, leading to an elevated risk of serious side effects such as myopathy (muscle weakness or pain) and rhabdomyolysis, a condition where muscle tissue breaks down and releases proteins into the bloodstream, potentially causing kidney damage. Therefore, when erythromycin is prescribed to patients taking statins, healthcare providers may need to adjust the statin dose or switch to a statin that is less dependent on CYP3A4 for metabolism, such as pravastatin.

Calcium Channel Blockers (Heart Medications): Calcium channel blockers, such as verapamil, diltiazem, and amlodipine, are commonly prescribed to treat high blood pressure, angina, and certain heart arrhythmias. Erythromycin can inhibit the metabolism of these medications by blocking CYP3A4, leading to elevated blood levels of the calcium channel blockers. This interaction can result in excessive lowering of blood pressure (hypotension) and an increased risk of side effects, such as dizziness, fainting, or even more severe cardiovascular issues like bradycardia (slow heart rate) or heart failure. Patients on calcium channel blockers should be closely monitored for signs of toxicity when starting erythromycin, and dose adjustments may be necessary.

Anticonvulsants (Anti-Seizure Medications): Certain anticonvulsants, such as carbamazepine and phenytoin, are metabolized by the CYP450 system. Erythromycin can increase the plasma levels of these drugs, leading to an increased risk of side effects such as dizziness, nausea, confusion, and, in severe cases, toxic reactions such as liver damage or blood disorders. Monitoring of drug levels and adjustments in the anticonvulsant dosage may be required to prevent toxicity when these medications are co-administered with erythromycin.

2. Cardiac Medications and Risk of QT Prolongation

Erythromycin has the potential to prolong the QT interval, which is the time taken for the heart's electrical system to recharge between beats, as measured on an electrocardiogram (ECG). QT prolongation can lead to a potentially fatal type of heart arrhythmia called *torsades de pointes*. When erythromycin is combined with other medications that also prolong the QT interval, the risk of developing this dangerous arrhythmia increases significantly.

Antiarrhythmic Medications: Antiarrhythmic drugs, such as amiodarone, sotalol, and quinidine, are used to treat irregular heart rhythms. These medications also have the potential to prolong the QT interval. Co-administration of erythromycin with antiarrhythmic drugs can lead to a compounded effect on the QT interval, significantly increasing the risk of torsades de pointes or other serious arrhythmias. Patients receiving both erythromycin and antiarrhythmics should be carefully monitored, and alternative antibiotics that do not affect the QT interval should be considered if possible.

Antipsychotics and Antidepressants: Some

antipsychotic and antidepressant medications, such as haloperidol, chlorpromazine, citalopram, and fluoxetine, are also associated with QT prolongation. When taken together with erythromycin, the combined effect can raise the risk of cardiac arrhythmias. Patients on these medications should be evaluated for their risk of QT prolongation before starting erythromycin. In cases where both drugs are necessary, ECG monitoring may be warranted to detect any abnormalities in the heart's electrical activity.

Diuretics: Certain diuretics, also known as water pills, can cause electrolyte imbalances, such as low potassium or magnesium levels, which increase the risk of QT prolongation when erythromycin is administered. Diuretics like furosemide or hydrochlorothiazide, when combined with erythromycin, can exacerbate the risk of arrhythmias. It is crucial to monitor electrolyte levels in patients who are on both erythromycin and diuretics to avoid complications related to low potassium or magnesium levels.

3. Interaction with Anticoagulants and Blood Thinners

Erythromycin can interact with anticoagulant medications, such as warfarin, which are used to prevent blood clots. Warfarin is metabolized through the CYP450 system, and erythromycin's inhibition of CYP3A4 can lead to increased warfarin levels in the blood. This interaction raises the risk of excessive bleeding, as warfarin's blood-thinning effects may become more potent.

Patients taking both erythromycin and warfarin should have their blood clotting time (measured as the international normalized ratio or INR) monitored more frequently to ensure that it remains within a safe range. If the INR becomes elevated, the warfarin dosage may need to be reduced to prevent the risk of dangerous bleeding events such as gastrointestinal bleeding, bruising, or hemorrhagic stroke.

4. Erythromycin and Immunosuppressants

Immunosuppressants, such as cyclosporine and tacrolimus, are medications used to prevent organ rejection after a transplant or to treat autoimmune diseases. These drugs are also metabolized by CYP3A4, and erythromycin's inhibition of this enzyme can lead to dangerously high levels of the immunosuppressants in the bloodstream. Elevated levels of cyclosporine or tacrolimus can cause kidney damage, increased susceptibility to infections, and other toxic effects.

Patients taking erythromycin in combination with immunosuppressants should have their blood levels of the immunosuppressant monitored closely to avoid toxicity. In some cases, the dose of the immunosuppressant may need to be reduced while the patient is on erythromycin.

5. Erythromycin and Gastrointestinal Medications

Erythromycin can interact with medications used to treat gastrointestinal conditions, such as proton pump inhibitors (PPIs) or drugs that affect gastric motility. Erythromycin itself acts as a prokinetic agent, stimulating the motility of the gastrointestinal tract by binding to motilin receptors. When combined with other drugs that affect gastric emptying or motility, such as metoclopramide, the effects can be amplified, leading to increased gastrointestinal side effects like cramping, diarrhea, or nausea.

Additionally, erythromycin can increase the absorption of certain medications that are affected by gastric pH or transit time through the digestive tract. For example, erythromycin may enhance the absorption of digoxin, a medication used to treat heart conditions. Increased levels of digoxin can lead to toxicity, characterized by symptoms such as nausea, vomiting, visual disturbances, and cardiac arrhythmias. Patients taking erythromycin and digoxin should be monitored for signs of digoxin toxicity, and dose adjustments may be necessary.

6. Erythromycin and Oral Hypoglycemics (Antidiabetic Drugs)

Erythromycin can interact with certain oral hypoglycemic medications used to treat diabetes, such as sulfonylureas. These medications lower blood sugar levels, and erythromycin may increase their effects by inhibiting their metabolism. This interaction can result in hypoglycemia (low blood sugar), a condition that can cause symptoms like shakiness, sweating, confusion, dizziness, and, in severe cases, loss of consciousness or seizures.

Patients with diabetes who are taking erythromycin alongside oral hypoglycemics should closely monitor their blood sugar levels to avoid hypoglycemia. Healthcare providers may need to adjust the dosage of the antidiabetic medication while the patient is on erythromycin.

Conclusion

Erythromycin's interactions with other medications can have significant clinical implications, primarily due to its ability to inhibit the CYP450 enzyme system and its effects on the heart and gastrointestinal tract. From increasing the risk of cardiac arrhythmias when combined with QT-prolonging drugs to raising the potential for toxicity with medications metabolized by CYP3A4, erythromycin requires careful consideration when used alongside other medications. Patients taking erythromycin should always provide their healthcare providers with a comprehensive list of their current medications to prevent harmful interactions, and they should be monitored for any signs of toxicity or adverse effects during treatment.

The end

www.ingramcontent.com/pod-product-compliance
Lightning Source LLC
Chambersburg PA
CBHW030050230526
45471CB00003B/1028